DR. LARRY GODSON

Gastritis-friendly Flavors

A Gastritis Healing Cookbook

Contents

1

Introduction

Welcome to "Gastritis-friendly Flavors," a cookbook designed to support individuals managing gastritis through delicious and soothing recipes. Gastritis, an inflammation of the stomach lining, can be alleviated with a thoughtful and nourishing diet. This cookbook aims to provide you with tasty and healing recipes that won't compromise on flavor.

If you or someone you know is navigating the challenges of gastritis, this cookbook is designed to be your culinary companion on the journey to better digestive health.

This cookbook aims to provide you with a diverse collection of recipes that not only adhere to gastritis-friendly guidelines but also celebrate the joy of eating. From soothing soups to satisfying main courses and delectable desserts, each recipe is crafted to be gentle on the stomach while maintaining the essence of deliciousness.Let's embark on a journey of culinary delight while taking care of your stomach health!

2

Understanding Gastritis

Gastritis is the inflammation of the stomach lining, a condition that can cause discomfort, pain, and other digestive issues. Understanding the causes and triggers of gastritis is crucial for managing and preventing flare-ups. In this chapter, we'll delve into the basics of gastritis, its symptoms, and how dietary choices can significantly impact your stomach health.

What is Gastritis?

Gastritis is characterized by the inflammation of the stomach lining, which can be acute or chronic. It is often caused by factors such as bacterial infections (Helicobacter pylori), long-term use of nonsteroidal anti-inflammatory drugs (NSAIDs), excessive alcohol consumption, stress, and autoimmune diseases.

Symptoms of Gastritis

Common symptoms of gastritis include abdominal pain, bloating, indigestion, nausea, and a burning sensation in the stomach. It's essential to recognize these signs to take timely action and make necessary dietary adjustments.

The Role of Diet in Gastritis Management

Diet plays a crucial role in managing and preventing gastritis. Certain foods and beverages can either exacerbate inflammation or contribute to the healing process. By understanding which ingredients to include and which to avoid, you can create a gastritis-friendly diet that supports your overall well-being.

Foods to Avoid with Gastritis

Some foods and beverages can irritate the stomach lining and should be limited or avoided. This includes spicy foods, acidic fruits, caffeinated and carbonated beverages, and high-fat or fried foods. Identifying and eliminating these triggers is vital for preventing flare-ups.

Foods That Soothe Gastritis

On the flip side, there are many foods that can soothe inflammation and promote healing. These include bland, easily digestible foods such as oats, bananas, lean proteins, and certain herbs. We'll explore these ingredients in detail throughout the cookbook.

Importance of Regular Meals

Establishing a regular eating schedule can help manage gastritis symptoms. Consuming smaller, more frequent meals throughout the day can prevent the stomach from becoming overly full, reducing the likelihood of irritation.

Hydration for Digestive Wellness

Staying hydrated is crucial for digestive health. We'll discuss the importance of water intake and explore soothing beverages like herbal teas that can contribute to overall stomach wellness.

As we move forward in this cookbook, keep these fundamental principles in mind. By understanding the dynamics of gastritis and the impact of dietary choices, you can make informed decisions to support your journey toward a healthier, happier stomach.

3

The Gastritis Pantry

To create gastritis-friendly meals, it's essential to stock your kitchen with ingredients that promote healing and soothe the stomach. In this chapter, we'll explore a comprehensive list of pantry staples, ensuring you have the necessary tools to craft delicious and gentle recipes.

Grains and Carbohydrates

Oats: A soothing and easily digestible grain that can be used for breakfast or in baking.

Quinoa: A protein-rich alternative to traditional grains, gentle on the stomach.

Brown Rice: An easily digestible whole grain that forms a versatile base for many dishes.

Lean Proteins

Chicken: Skinless, boneless chicken breasts or thighs are a lean source of protein.

Turkey: Ground turkey or turkey breast is another low-fat protein option.

Fish: Choose easily digestible fish like salmon or cod for omega-3 fatty acids.

Tofu: A plant-based protein source suitable for various dishes.

Fruits and Vegetables

Bananas: An easily digestible fruit that can be a go-to snack or breakfast ingredient.

Apples: Particularly helpful for baked desserts and snacks.

Leafy Greens: Spinach and kale offer essential nutrients without being too harsh on the stomach.

Carrots: A versatile and gentle root vegetable.

Herbs and Spices

Fresh Herbs: Mint, basil, and parsley add flavor without causing irritation.

Ginger: Known for its anti-inflammatory properties and soothing effect on the stomach.

Turmeric: Contains curcumin, which may help reduce inflammation.

Fats and Oils

Olive Oil: A heart-healthy oil that can be used for sautéing and dressing.

Coconut Oil: Provides a flavorful alternative for cooking and baking.

Avocado: A nutrient-rich source of healthy fats.

Dairy and Non-Dairy Alternatives

Greek Yogurt: A probiotic-rich option that can support gut health.

Almond Milk: A dairy-free alternative that can be used in various recipes.

Beverages

Herbal Teas: Chamomile, peppermint, and ginger teas can be soothing on the stomach.

Water: Staying hydrated is crucial for digestive wellness.

Condiments and Flavor Enhancers

Honey: A natural sweetener that can be used in moderation.

Low-acidic Mustard: Adds flavor without causing irritation.

Apple Cider Vinegar: While acidic, some find it beneficial in small quantities; use with caution.

By maintaining a well-stocked gastritis-friendly pantry, you'll have the foundation for creating nourishing meals that support your stomach health. As we move forward in the cookbook, these ingredients will come together to form delicious and healing recipes.

4

Breakfasts to Start Your Day Right

Breakfast is often considered the most important meal of the day, and for those managing gastritis, it's an opportunity to kickstart your morning with gentle and soothing options. In this chapter, we'll explore a variety of breakfast recipes that are not only delicious but also easy on the stomach.

Soothing Oatmeal Bowl

Ingredients:

- 1/2 cup rolled oats
- 1 cup almond milk (or any non-dairy alternative)
- 1 ripe banana, mashed
- 1 tablespoon honey (optional)
- 1/2 teaspoon ground cinnamon
- Toppings: Sliced banana, a sprinkle of chia seeds

Instructions:

1. In a saucepan, combine rolled oats and almond milk. Cook over medium heat, stirring occasionally, until the oats are soft and have absorbed the liquid.

2. Stir in the mashed banana, honey (if using), and ground cinnamon.

3. Cook for an additional 2-3 minutes until the mixture reaches your desired consistency.

4. Pour the oatmeal into a bowl and top with sliced banana and chia seeds.

Greek Yogurt Parfait

Ingredients:

- 1 cup Greek yogurt
- 1/2 cup granola (ensure it's low in added sugars)
- 1/2 cup mixed berries (blueberries, strawberries)
- 1 tablespoon honey

Instructions:

1. In a glass or bowl, layer Greek yogurt, granola, and mixed berries.
2. Repeat the layers until you reach the top.
3. Drizzle honey over the parfait and serve chilled.

Banana and Almond Butter Toast

Ingredients:

- 2 slices whole grain bread
- 2 tablespoons almond butter
- 1 ripe banana, sliced

Instructions:

1. Toast the whole grain bread slices.
2. Spread almond butter evenly on each slice.
3. Top with sliced banana.
4. For added sweetness, drizzle a touch of honey.

Chia Seed Pudding

Ingredients:

- 1/4 cup chia seeds
- 1 cup almond milk
- 1/2 teaspoon vanilla extract
- Fresh berries for topping

Instructions:

1. In a bowl, mix chia seeds, almond milk, and vanilla extract.
2. Refrigerate for at least 2 hours or overnight, allowing the chia seeds to absorb the liquid.
3. Stir well before serving and top with fresh berries.

Smoothie Bowl

Ingredients:

- 1 frozen banana
- 1/2 cup frozen mixed berries
- 1/2 cup spinach leaves
- 1/2 cup almond milk
- Toppings: Sliced kiwi, coconut flakes, and a sprinkle of granola

Instructions:

1. Blend the frozen banana, mixed berries, spinach, and almond milk until smooth.

2. Pour the smoothie into a bowl and add your favorite toppings.

These breakfast recipes are designed to be gentle on the stomach while providing the nutrients and energy needed to start your day on a positive note. Feel free to customize these recipes based on your preferences and dietary needs.

5

Soothing Soups and Stews

When managing gastritis, incorporating soothing and easy-to-digest soups and stews into your diet can provide comfort and essential nutrients. In this chapter, we'll explore a variety of recipes designed to be gentle on the stomach while offering delicious flavors.

Healing Chicken Broth

Ingredients:

- 2 boneless, skinless chicken breasts
- 8 cups water
- 2 carrots, peeled and chopped
- 2 celery stalks, chopped
- 1 onion, quartered
- 2 cloves garlic, crushed
- 1 teaspoon fresh ginger, grated
- Salt and pepper to taste
- Fresh parsley for garnish

Instructions:

1. In a large pot, combine chicken breasts, water, carrots, celery, onion, garlic, and ginger.

2. Bring to a boil, then reduce heat and simmer for 1-2 hours.

3. Remove chicken, shred it, and return it to the pot.

4. Season with salt and pepper to taste.

5. Garnish with fresh parsley before serving.

Quinoa and Vegetable Stew

Ingredients:

- 1 cup quinoa, rinsed
- 4 cups vegetable broth
- 1 tablespoon olive oil
- 1 onion, diced
- 2 carrots, sliced
- 2 celery stalks, chopped
- 1 bell pepper, diced
- 2 cloves garlic, minced
- 1 teaspoon dried thyme
- Salt and pepper to taste
- Fresh parsley for garnish

Instructions:

1. In a pot, heat olive oil over medium heat. Add onion, carrots, celery, bell pepper, and garlic. Sauté until vegetables are softened.

2. Add quinoa and vegetable broth. Bring to a boil, then reduce heat and simmer for 15-20 minutes or until quinoa is cooked.

3. Season with thyme, salt, and pepper.

4. Garnish with fresh parsley before serving.

Butternut Squash and Ginger Soup

Ingredients:

- 1 medium-sized butternut squash, peeled and cubed
- 1 tablespoon olive oil
- 1 onion, chopped
- 2 cloves garlic, minced
- 1 tablespoon fresh ginger, grated
- 4 cups vegetable broth
- Salt and pepper to taste

- Coconut milk for garnish

Instructions:

1. In a large pot, heat olive oil over medium heat. Add onion, garlic, and ginger. Sauté until fragrant.

2. Add butternut squash and vegetable broth. Bring to a boil, then reduce heat and simmer until the squash is tender.

3. Use an immersion blender to puree the soup until smooth.

4. Season with salt and pepper.

5. Serve with a drizzle of coconut milk.

Lentil and Spinach Soup

Ingredients:

- 1 cup dried green lentils, rinsed
- 6 cups vegetable broth
- 1 tablespoon olive oil
- 1 onion, diced
- 2 carrots, sliced
- 2 celery stalks, chopped
- 2 cloves garlic, minced
- 1 teaspoon cumin
- 1 teaspoon coriander
- Salt and pepper to taste
- Fresh spinach leaves

Instructions:

1. In a pot, heat olive oil over medium heat. Add onion, carrots, celery, and garlic. Sauté until vegetables are softened.

2. Add lentils, vegetable broth, cumin, coriander, salt, and pepper. Bring to a boil, then reduce heat and simmer until lentils are cooked.

3. Add fresh spinach leaves and cook until wilted.

4. Adjust seasoning before serving.

These soothing soup and stew recipes are designed to be easy on the stomach while providing essential nutrients. Experiment with different combinations and adjust seasoning according to your taste preferences.

6

Light and Nutrient-packed Salads

Salads can be a refreshing and nutritious addition to your gastritis-friendly diet. In this chapter, we'll explore creative combinations of ingredients that not only soothe your stomach but also tantalize your taste buds. These salads are light, flavorful, and packed with essential nutrients.

Grilled Chicken and Mixed Greens Salad

Ingredients:
- 2 boneless, skinless chicken breasts
- Mixed salad greens (e.g., spinach, arugula, and romaine)
- Cherry tomatoes, halved
- Cucumber, sliced
- Avocado, diced
- Olive oil and lemon dressing (olive oil, lemon juice, salt, and pepper)

Instructions:
1. Grill chicken breasts until fully cooked, then slice into thin strips.
2. In a large bowl, combine mixed greens, cherry tomatoes, cucumber, and avocado.
3. Top with grilled chicken strips.
4. Drizzle with olive oil and lemon dressing.

Quinoa and Vegetable Salad

Ingredients:

- 1 cup cooked quinoa

- Mixed vegetables (bell peppers, cherry tomatoes, cucumber)

- Fresh herbs (mint, parsley)

- Feta cheese, crumbled (optional)

- Balsamic vinaigrette dressing

Instructions:

1. In a large bowl, combine cooked quinoa, mixed vegetables, and fresh herbs.

2. Toss with balsamic vinaigrette dressing.

3. Top with crumbled feta cheese if desired.

Citrus Shrimp and Avocado Salad

Ingredients:

- Shrimp, peeled and deveined

- Mixed salad greens

- Avocado, sliced

- Orange segments

- Red onion, thinly sliced

- Cilantro for garnish

- Citrus vinaigrette dressing

Instructions:

1. Sauté shrimp until cooked through.

2. In a large bowl, combine mixed greens, avocado, orange segments, and red onion.

3. Top with cooked shrimp.

4. Drizzle with citrus vinaigrette dressing and garnish with cilantro.

Spinach and Strawberry Salad

Ingredients:

- Baby spinach leaves

- Fresh strawberries, sliced

- Goat cheese, crumbled

- Walnuts, chopped
- Balsamic glaze dressing

Instructions:

1. In a bowl, combine baby spinach, sliced strawberries, crumbled goat cheese, and chopped walnuts.

2. Drizzle with balsamic glaze dressing and toss gently.

Mediterranean Chickpea Salad

Ingredients:

- Canned chickpeas, rinsed and drained
- Cherry tomatoes, halved
- Cucumber, diced
- Kalamata olives, pitted and sliced
- Red onion, finely chopped
- Feta cheese, crumbled
- Olive oil and lemon dressing

Instructions:

1. In a large bowl, combine chickpeas, cherry tomatoes, cucumber, olives, red onion, and feta cheese.

2. Drizzle with olive oil and lemon dressing, tossing to coat.

These salads offer a delightful mix of textures and flavors while being gentle on the stomach. Experiment with different combinations and dressings to find your favorite gastritis–friendly salad recipes.

7

Wholesome Mains for Satisfying Meals

Creating gastritis-friendly main courses doesn't mean sacrificing flavor or satisfaction. In this chapter, we'll explore hearty and nutritious recipes that are easy on the stomach, ensuring that you can enjoy satisfying meals without compromising your digestive health.

Baked Salmon with Lemon and Dill

Ingredients:

- Salmon fillets
- Fresh lemon slices
- Fresh dill, chopped
- Olive oil
- Salt and pepper to taste

Instructions:

1. Preheat the oven to 375°F (190°C).
2. Place salmon fillets on a baking sheet lined with parchment paper.
3. Drizzle olive oil over the salmon, season with salt and pepper, and top with lemon slices and chopped dill.
4. Bake for 15-20 minutes or until the salmon is cooked through.

Quinoa and Vegetable Stir-Fry

Ingredients:

- 1 cup cooked quinoa
- Mixed vegetables (bell peppers, broccoli, carrots)
- Tofu or chicken, diced
- Soy sauce or tamari
- Sesame oil
- Garlic, minced
- Ginger, grated

Instructions:

1. In a wok or large skillet, heat sesame oil over medium heat.

2. Add tofu or chicken and cook until browned.

3. Add mixed vegetables, garlic, and ginger. Stir-fry until vegetables are tender.

4. Stir in cooked quinoa and soy sauce or tamari. Cook for an additional 2-3 minutes.

Turkey and Sweet Potato Skillet

Ingredients:

- Ground turkey
- Sweet potatoes, peeled and diced
- Onion, chopped
- Garlic, minced
- Paprika
- Cumin
- Salt and pepper to taste
- Fresh cilantro for garnish

Instructions:

1. In a large skillet, cook ground turkey until browned.

2. Add sweet potatoes, onion, and garlic. Cook until sweet potatoes are tender.

3. Season with paprika, cumin, salt, and pepper.

4. Garnish with fresh cilantro before serving.

Ginger and Garlic Baked Chicken

Ingredients:

- Chicken thighs or breasts
- Fresh ginger, grated
- Garlic, minced
- Soy sauce or tamari
- Honey
- Olive oil
- Sesame seeds for garnish

Instructions:

1. Preheat the oven to 400°F (200°C).
2. In a bowl, mix grated ginger, minced garlic, soy sauce or tamari, honey, and olive oil.
3. Place chicken in a baking dish and pour the marinade over it.
4. Bake for 25-30 minutes or until the chicken is cooked through.
5. Garnish with sesame seeds before serving.

Veggie and Brown Rice Stuffed Bell Peppers

Ingredients:

- Bell peppers, halved and cleaned
- Brown rice, cooked
- Black beans, drained and rinsed
- Corn kernels
- Cherry tomatoes, halved
- Cumin, chili powder, salt, and pepper to taste
- Shredded cheese for topping (optional)

Instructions:

1. Preheat the oven to 375°F (190°C).
2. In a bowl, mix cooked brown rice, black beans, corn, cherry tomatoes, and seasonings.
3. Stuff bell peppers with the rice mixture and place them in a baking dish.
4. Bake for 20-25 minutes. If desired, top with shredded cheese in the last 5 minutes of baking.

These wholesome main courses are designed to be gentle on the stomach while offering a satisfying and flavorful dining experience. Enjoy experimenting with different protein sources and seasonings to tailor these recipes to your taste preferences.

8

Snacks for Sensitive Stomachs

Maintaining energy levels throughout the day without irritating your stomach is crucial when managing gastritis. In this chapter, we'll explore a variety of snacks that are not only gentle on the stomach but also delicious and satisfying. These snacks can be enjoyed between meals or as a small treat to curb hunger.

Homemade Granola Bars

Ingredients:

- 1 cup old-fashioned oats
- 1/2 cup nuts (almonds, walnuts), chopped
- 1/4 cup honey or maple syrup
- 1/4 cup nut butter (almond, peanut)
- 1/2 cup dried fruit (raisins, cranberries)
- 1/4 teaspoon vanilla extract

Instructions:

1. In a bowl, combine oats, chopped nuts, honey or maple syrup, nut butter, dried fruit, and vanilla extract.

2. Press the mixture into a lined baking dish and refrigerate for at least 2 hours.

3. Once set, cut into bars and enjoy.

Roasted Chickpeas

Ingredients:

- 1 can chickpeas, drained and rinsed
- 1 tablespoon olive oil
- Seasonings (paprika, cumin, garlic powder, salt)

Instructions:

1. Preheat the oven to 400°F (200°C).
2. Pat chickpeas dry with a paper towel.
3. Toss chickpeas in olive oil and seasonings.
4. Spread them on a baking sheet and roast for 20-25 minutes or until crispy.

Greek Yogurt with Berries

Ingredients:

- Greek yogurt
- Mixed berries (blueberries, strawberries)
- Honey for drizzling (optional)

Instructions:

1. Spoon Greek yogurt into a bowl.
2. Top with mixed berries.
3. Drizzle with honey if desired.

Rice Cakes with Almond Butter and Banana

Ingredients:

- Rice cakes
- Almond butter
- Banana, sliced

Instructions:

1. Spread almond butter on rice cakes.
2. Top with banana slices.

Nut and Seed Trail Mix

Ingredients:

- Almonds, walnuts, pumpkin seeds, sunflower seeds
- Dried fruit (apricots, figs)

- Dark chocolate chips

Instructions:

1. Mix all ingredients in a bowl.

2. Portion into small snack-sized bags for convenience.

Cottage Cheese with Pineapple

Ingredients:

- Cottage cheese

- Fresh pineapple, diced

Instructions:

1. Spoon cottage cheese into a bowl.

2. Top with fresh pineapple.

These snacks offer a balance of protein, fiber, and healthy fats to keep you satisfied between meals. Feel free to customize the recipes based on your preferences and dietary needs.

9

Desserts without the Discomfort

Satisfying your sweet tooth while managing gastritis is possible with desserts that are gentle on the stomach. In this chapter, we'll explore a variety of delicious and soothing desserts that won't trigger inflammation and can be enjoyed in moderation.

Baked Apples with Cinnamon
   Ingredients:
   - Apples, cored and halved
   - Cinnamon
   - Honey (optional)
   - Chopped nuts (almonds, walnuts)

   Instructions:
   1. Preheat the oven to 375°F (190°C).
   2. Place cored and halved apples on a baking sheet.
   3. Sprinkle with cinnamon and drizzle with honey if desired.
   4. Bake for 20-25 minutes or until apples are tender.
   5. Top with chopped nuts before serving.

Banana Muffins
   Ingredients:
   - Ripe bananas, mashed

- Eggs
- Almond flour
- Baking powder
- Cinnamon
- Vanilla extract
- Chopped dark chocolate (optional)

Instructions:

1. Preheat the oven to 350°F (175°C) and line a muffin tin with paper liners.

2. In a bowl, mix mashed bananas, eggs, almond flour, baking powder, cinnamon, and vanilla extract.

3. Fold in chopped dark chocolate if using.

4. Spoon the batter into muffin cups and bake for 20-25 minutes or until a toothpick comes out clean.

Chia Seed Pudding with Berries

Ingredients:

- Chia seeds
- Almond milk
- Vanilla extract
- Mixed berries

Instructions:

1. In a jar, mix chia seeds, almond milk, and vanilla extract.

2. Refrigerate for at least 2 hours or overnight, stirring occasionally.

3. Layer the chia pudding with mixed berries before serving.

Pumpkin Smoothie Bowl

Ingredients:

- Pumpkin puree
- Frozen banana
- Greek yogurt
- Pumpkin spice (cinnamon, nutmeg, ginger)
- Granola for topping

Instructions:

1. Blend pumpkin puree, frozen banana, Greek yogurt, and pumpkin spice until smooth.

2. Pour into a bowl and top with granola.

Almond Flour Cookies

Ingredients:

- Almond flour
- Coconut oil
- Maple syrup
- Vanilla extract
- Dark chocolate chips (optional)

Instructions:

1. Preheat the oven to 350°F (175°C) and line a baking sheet with parchment paper.

2. In a bowl, mix almond flour, melted coconut oil, maple syrup, and vanilla extract.

3. Fold in dark chocolate chips if using.

4. Drop spoonfuls of dough onto the baking sheet and bake for 10–12 minutes or until edges are golden.

Mango Sorbet

Ingredients:

- Frozen mango chunks
- Coconut water
- Lime juice
- Mint leaves for garnish

Instructions:

1. Blend frozen mango chunks, coconut water, and lime juice until smooth.

2. Scoop into bowls and garnish with fresh mint leaves.

These desserts offer a sweet treat without causing discomfort. Remember to enjoy them in moderation and listen to your body's response. Feel free to customize these recipes to suit your taste preferences and dietary needs.

10

Beverages for Digestive Harmony

Hydrating with soothing and digestive-friendly beverages is an integral part of managing gastritis. In this chapter, we'll explore a variety of drinks that not only keep you hydrated but also contribute to digestive wellness.

Herbal Teas

Options:

- Chamomile Tea: Known for its calming and anti-inflammatory properties.

- Peppermint Tea: Can help soothe the digestive tract.

- Ginger Tea: Contains compounds that may reduce inflammation.

Instructions:

1. Choose your preferred herbal tea bag or loose leaves.

2. Steep in hot water for 5-7 minutes.

3. Sweeten with honey if desired.

Infused Water

Options:

- Cucumber and Mint Infused Water: Refreshing and hydrating.

- Lemon and Basil Infused Water: Adds a burst of flavor without acidity.

- Berry and Citrus Infused Water: Packed with antioxidants.

Instructions:

1. Add sliced fruits, vegetables, and herbs to a pitcher of water.

2. Refrigerate for at least 2 hours before serving.

Golden Turmeric Latte

Ingredients:

- Turmeric powder

- Almond milk

- Honey

- Cinnamon

Instructions:

1. In a saucepan, heat almond milk over medium heat.

2. Whisk in turmeric powder, honey, and a pinch of cinnamon.

3. Heat until warm but not boiling. Whisk continuously.

4. Pour into a mug and enjoy.

Aloe Vera Juice Smoothie

Ingredients:

- Aloe vera juice (pure, without added sugars)

- Pineapple chunks

- Banana

- Coconut water

Instructions:

1. Blend aloe vera juice, pineapple chunks, banana, and coconut water until smooth.

2. Pour into a glass and savor the tropical goodness.

Carrot and Ginger Juice

Ingredients:

- Carrots, peeled and chopped

- Fresh ginger, grated

- Apple, cored and chopped

- Water

Instructions:

1. Juice carrots, ginger, and apple.

2. Dilute with water if needed.

3. Serve over ice for a refreshing beverage.

Minty Iced Green Tea

Ingredients:

- Green tea bags

- Fresh mint leaves

- Lemon slices

- Ice cubes

Instructions:

1. Steep green tea bags in hot water and let it cool.

2. Add fresh mint leaves, lemon slices, and ice cubes.

3. Stir and enjoy a cooling iced tea.

Staying hydrated with these digestive-friendly beverages can complement your gastritis-friendly diet. Experiment with different flavors and combinations to find the drinks that soothe your stomach and suit your taste preferences.

11

Conclusion

As we conclude our gastritis-friendly cookbook, we hope this culinary journey has provided you with a delightful array of recipes that nourish your body without compromising on flavor. Managing gastritis doesn't mean sacrificing the joy of eating; rather, it invites us to explore new ingredients and cooking methods that promote healing and digestive wellness.

In this cookbook, we've covered a range of meals, from breakfast to dessert, and beverages designed to support your digestive health. From the healing properties of ginger in soups to the soothing effects of herbal teas, each recipe has been thoughtfully crafted to be gentle on the stomach while delivering a satisfying culinary experience.

Remember that everyone's body responds differently, so it's essential to pay attention to how your stomach reacts to different foods. Feel free to customize these recipes based on your taste preferences, dietary restrictions, and specific needs.

As you continue on your gastritis-friendly journey, consider maintaining a food journal to track what works best for you. Gradually reintroduce foods, and consult with a healthcare professional or a nutritionist for personalized guidance.

Cooking for gastritis is not just about restriction; it's an opportunity to explore new flavors, nourish your body, and cultivate a positive relationship with food. Here's to good health, happy digestion, and the joy of savoring delicious, gastritis-friendly meals!

Yours sincerely

Dr. Larry Godson